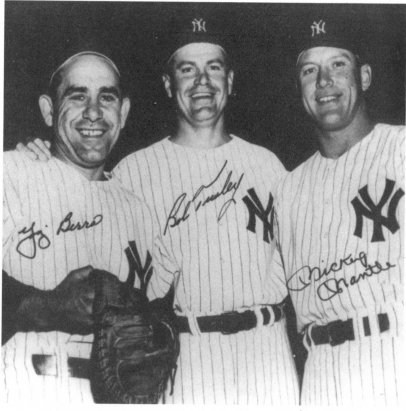

Yogi Berra   Bob Turley   Mickey Mantle

The Crow
And The Eagle
A True Fable

by
John K Danenbarger

Published by
Stormblock Publishing
1 Broad Street, Suite 9
Salem, MA 01970
USA

Design and Illustrations
William Cloutman

Library of Congress Control Number: 2003101396

International Standard Book Number (ISBN): 0-9728998-0-4

Printed in the United States of America

First Printing

Acknowledgments

I want to thank my wife for all the knowledge, forbearance, and understanding she offered for the creation of this book. She introduced me to Bob Turley. As we became friends, I realized Bob's wisdom needed to be passed on not only to his own people, but to anyone who wants to succeed through fair play.

While I wanted to thank Bob for his patience through all the time he spent with me, Bob wanted to take it a step further and said, "When Sandy Weill's company merged with us, it was the best thing that could have happened to my business ... because of Sandy...his toughness, his integrity." I think Bob was buoyed to find such a rare bird of his own feather in Sandy.

The news headlines report disaster, crime, and blood. ("If it bleeds, it leads.") A good airplane flight is never a headline any more than great leadership. But both of these gentlemen are examples of how business can be run with integrity, making it a joy for me to write this book based on Bob Turley's persona and to share his insight with you.

John K Danenbarger

PART ONE
Feather Tale

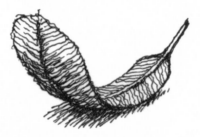

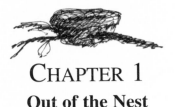

CHAPTER 1
Out of the Nest

A crow and an eagle sat hidden in a large elm deep in the woods because the crow didn't want to be caught talking to an eagle. It just wouldn't look right. So with the sharp vision that eagles have, the eagle kept a lookout.

The crow was nervous. "Why did you want to see me?" he asked, as he scratched under a wing.

"I need to talk with you," said the eagle. "Sometimes it gets lonely at the top."

"Don't get sarcastic with me," said the crow.

"Okay. I was joking. But I do have a good reason. Just quit being so nervous."

The crow eyed the eagle with suspicion. "It's in my nature."

"Maybe you should trust those of a feather."

"You ain't my feather," the crow snapped.

"Are you sure?" asked the eagle.

"Come ooooon! I thought you eagles had vision."

"Exactly!" said the eagle.

"Look atcha," said the crow. "Fine feathers. Elegant stance. Proud beak. I don't know what I'm doing in the same tree with ya."

"I used to be a crow," said the eagle, looking the crow right in the eye.

The crow said "Gawk!" and couldn't stop "gawking." He fluttered up and down and nearly fell off the branch.

"Take it easy," said the eagle. "You will attract a crowd. Just take it easy."

Continuing to fake bad English, the crow said, "Well, we crows is smart so don't go telling me you was a crow, or I'm leaving."

"I *was* once. I thought I was like every other bird. Incidentally, just call me Bob."

"I'll make you bob *and* duck if you don't stop screwing around with me. I'm leavin'."

"No, wait. Real crows have curiosity. Don't *you*?"

"Well, whaduwant?" said the crow.

"I want your success," said the eagle. The crow was a little baffled by that statement and turned his head seeming to measure how far he would fall. Bob, the eagle, continued. "I have watched how you can outsmart the other crows and dominate the other birds, which is not always the nicest thing to do, but it gets the job done. In your case, feeding your family. But *barely* feeding your family. There is so much more."

"More what?" asked the crow.

"That is for you to discover. But wouldn't it be nice to be able to choose more than basic survival...claw to beak, so to speak?"

"Like what?"

"*That* is what I want to talk to you about. It is not easy for me to tell you what. It is something you need to discover, like the first time you were to leave the nest. Your parents couldn't *tell* you what it was like to fly. You just needed to know it was possible to fly and then do it. Right now, you don't know what *is* possible."

"Look. I got a nestful to feed. I don't have all day. I just can't afford to sit around squawking with you for hours."

"So spend a half-hour with me each day for a few days and I will open some skies for you."

"I'm pretty happy as it is," said the crow. "I know what I have. One day it may get better."

"Do you know what the definition of insanity is?" asked the eagle.

"Okay, tell me."

"It is the act of doing the same thing over and over and expecting change."

The crow twisted his head one way and then the other, seemingly deep in thought. Then he said, "I'll see you tomorrow."

"Okay," said the eagle. "Tomorrow, right here in this oak."

"This ain't no oak. This here is an *elm*," said the crow.

"Oops, your right," said the eagle. "Trees are not my strong point."

CHAPTER 2

Gawk Can't

"Look," said the crow. "I've been thinking about it. This is for the birds. I am a crow. You're an eagle. Eagles soar. Crows scavenge. We scrape the bottom of the barrel. Nothing can change that. I'll think about it. Maybe in the future."

"It is interesting you say that," said the eagle. "The future is the most expensive luxury in the world.[1] It is the period of time in which our affairs prosper, our friends are true, and our happiness assured.[2] Let me tell you a fairy tale about humans."

[1] Thornton Wilder
[2] Ambrose Bierce

It is hard to smile with a beak, but the crow seemed to smile at the idea. He loved fairy tales. "Once upon a time there was a boy named...oh, let's call him Bob, like me."

"He doesn't have a last name?" asked the crow.

"Yeah. Turley. He grew up in East Saint Louis, Illinois, with no special advantages. He was essentially just one of the flock. A boy among boys."

"When was this?" asked the crow.

"This was just around and after World War Two. So the economy wasn't that good and besides, his family wasn't rich. So, as I said, he was, and could have continued to be, just one of the many. He could have been afraid to be different.

"But what made him a little different was that he played baseball and loved it. He was so poor that he was lucky to have a glove, and he certainly had no uniform. He and some other boys played in the schoolyard, and everywhere else they could find, with broken bats and taped baseballs.

"Then just when Pearl Harbor was bombed...and he was eleven years old, the Junior Chamber of Commerce in town got a few businesses to form a baseball league. It was just a league of four teams with different age groups. Bob played the B-league for Burke Funeral Home. It was the proudest day of his life when the coach said, 'You made it' and handed him his uniform. He never forgot that day."

The crow said, "So what position did he play?"

"Pitcher, third base, and outfield. He was an excellent pitcher because most of his childhood he would throw things...

apples and rocks... that he found in his back yard. But in this league, he was only allowed to pitch a few innings. He was a good hitter and the coach wanted him to play, so he rotated Bob around in three positions."

"So he liked baseball."

"Oh, Bob loved sports. He played every sport there was around there...football, basketball. That was his entertainment. The church had the basketball team and made the condition that he could play on the team only if he went to church once a week. Bob now believes that the combination of the Rosemont Baptist Church and sports may have kept him and others from going the wrong way."

"Didn't he have any parents?"

"His dad was in the military at war and earning nothing. His mother had to work all the time, but she did come to all his games and showed her pride even if she didn't understand the game."

"So he wasn't an orphan."

"No, in fact, he feels that if parents only show interest in what their children are doing as his mother did, it is better than having the best school teacher in the whole world. So put all that together, he looks back and thinks he was fairly happy despite their relative poverty."

"Okay, fine. So what's so special?"

"He became a star with the best team in baseball history," said the eagle calmly, watching for the crow's reaction.

"He did?"

"Yep."

"All of a sudden?"

"Of course not, birdbrain. And *that* is just the point I want to make today. What is it in this boy that moved him out of a common neighborhood and made him different from the other kids in town?"

"Yeah, what?" The crow lifted one foot and then the other in impatience.

"So you want to know?"

"Yeah. Yeah," said the crow bobbing up and down.

"And why do you think that is?"

"Why what is?" asked the crow.

"You like this guy, don't you? He's like you. Scrappy. Bottom of the barrel."

"Yeah. So how'd he do it?"

"He wanted it," said the eagle.

"Come ooooon!" said the crow.

"He did. He wanted it bad. Even at a young age, he had started to believe in himself. He started to see himself out on the ball field of major league stadiums."

"You mean from playing three positions on a Chamber of Commerce team, he saw this?"

"Well, not right away. But in him was a competitive desire to win. For example, his sophomore year in high school he was told by the coach that the team was pretty well set, but, if Bob wanted, Bob could stick around for pitching and batting practice, but he would get no uniform. So instead of going along with that, Bob played in the city league. The coach was umpire in the city league and, when he saw Bob pitch, he asked him to help out the high school team the next year."

Anticipating, the crow said, "So he did."

"No, because he wasn't promised to play. So Bob stayed in the muni league. Finally in his senior year, the coach said Bob could pitch for the high school team. At the end of that year the Saint Louis Browns were in East Saint Louis and sent over a scout. When he was asked who the best ball player was, the coach said it was Bob. Bob was asked to try out for the Browns."

"And?" the crow said impatiently.

"Well, before we go any further, what do you think made him different from the rest of the flock so far?"

"He was really good," said the crow.

"Good at what?" asked the eagle.

"Baseball, stupid."

"But what made him good?"

"How do I know? He was just good. He was a natural ... I don't know."

"There are *millions* born every day with huge talent, but you would never know," said the eagle. "But to continue, Bob did sign with the Browns right after high school, went to the beginning day as a professional baseball player earning $200 a month for three months pitching Class D ball at Belleville, Illinois State League...and happy as a lark. He pitched nine wins and three losses. He got a $600 bonus and made $1,200 that year. The next year in 1949, he was sent to Aberdeen, South

Dakota to play class C league and earn $200 more that year. His pitching record was 25 wins and 3 losses."

The crow's beak fell open. "Wow. That's good."

"It's a record never to be beaten. And he started and finished every game, never to be taken out. Plus he had a 308 batting average."

"So the big boys wanted him, right?" said the crow.

"Actually, you're right. At the end of the '49 season he was asked to come up to the Saint Louis Browns to work out with them, and then for spring training, he went to Burbank, California, and stayed at the Hollywood Plaza Hotel on Hollywood and Vine."

"Ooo! Big time! He started meeting famous people and babes, I bet."

"Well, yes and no...sort of. Right across the street from the hotel was a camera shop where he loved to hang out because there was a hilarious guy who worked there by the name of Jerry Lewis."

"The Jerry Lewis?"

"Oh, yeah, but he wasn't known yet. And other times he saw famous people in nightclubs, but with his income, Bob couldn't afford to be there or take a date there. Not that he didn't want to. But he was neither rich nor famous. Nor did he drink."

"How boring," said the crow.

"You think so?" said the eagle. "Here is a boy going on twenty years and is now in the major leagues. Why do you think *he* was there at that level and not his other high school classmates who had also played baseball?"

"There you go again," said the crow. "How do I know?"

"Try to think about it."

"Well," said the crow, fluffing up, "you said something about his wanting it. I want lots of things, but I can't have them."

"You can't? Why not?"

The crow shook his head rapidly. "I don't know. I just know I can't."

The eagle was silent for a moment, staring eagle-eyed at the crow. Then he said, "A pessimist is someone who burns his bridges before he gets to them. John Lennon said it perfectly when he said, 'We ourselves are the people our mothers warned us against.' How do you think 'I know I can't' sounds? Do you think maybe you sound *just* like the other boys in Bob's class?"

"Huh?"

"Or do you think Bob thought he couldn't? That he was *too* poor and dumb?" said the eagle.

"No, of course, he didn't."

"How did he think?" asked the eagle.

"That he was good."

"That he was a good boy?" asked the eagle.

"Maybe so," said the crow, "but that is not what got him to the majors,"

"You are right," said the eagle. "So what did he think that made him get there?"

"That he could play ball."

The eagle paused again. "Don't you think his high

school teammates also thought they could play ball?"

The crow fluttered to another branch and back again in exasperation. "What do you want me to say?"

"Just put yourself on that high school field. Don't you think that there were at least one or two others on that team that were talented...maybe even more so than Bob? Maybe they even got to play on the high school team before Bob."

"So you want me to say he wanted it more."

"I don't want you to say anything. 'Wanting it more' comes from *something* and you need to know what that is."

"Yeah, what is it?"

"Think about when the coach told Bob that he couldn't play on the team. Bob could hang around, the coach said, but no uniform for him. What did Bob do?"

"Yeah, I heard you. He played city ball."

"Why did he do that? Why didn't he want to hang around with the other boys in his school? Most kids would have. What made him take the initiative to go play with adults in the city system?"

The crow said, "Gawk!" Then he flew off at top speed, leaving the eagle to squint after him.

CHAPTER 3
Walking Birds

The eagle wasn't sure that the crow would show up the next day, but the crow did. And immediately the crow said, as if he had never left, "I know why Bob made it to the majors." The eagle waited. The crow leaned forward and wiped both sides of his beak on the branch. "He made it because he knew he could. He saw himself there."

"Crow," said the eagle. "I picked you out of the flock because I knew you had something. Part of that something is brains. That is right. The problem with the other classmates in high school was that *they*, for whatever reason, did not see themselves as major league players. They either did not want to be major baseball players because they had other visions or they simply were incapable of seeing themselves as being major league."

The crow preened his feathers. "But Bob knew."

"Yes," said the eagle. "Bob knew. It wasn't even a question in his mind."

"And so he became a superstar and lived happily ever after. What's that got to do with me?" asked the crow.

"No, he didn't."

"So he became a drunk and failed his family and society," said the crow with a smirk.

"No, he didn't. Life had just begun and he had a lot of hard knocks to experience, as we all do."

"So get on with it. He made it to the big leagues. That must be it...everything he wanted."

"Crow, I thought you were smart," said the eagle, frowning an eagle frown. "Look. He *did* attain his dream, so then he needed to create new goals...new visions. If his goal stayed what it was...just to play baseball in the major leagues, and he was happy with that, then his next position would have been to sell hotdogs. He needed to picture himself as a winner in this new huge competition of major league baseball players...from all over the United States and who all arrived in this elite situation because they believed that they could get there. Bob was no longer competing with high school kids. He was now competing with hundreds of winners, and he was the green rookie. You understand, Crow?"

"Gawk!"

"And now *nobody* really cared whether he succeeded,

except his mother and him. At that level of sports, there is so much competition that it is simply up to the individual player to know and decide if he or she is going to have further success. Nobody is babying them, coddling them, or even pushing them. The team management decides (and, at that time, even more so) who is going to be on the team and the coach sets up the strategy. The good coaches do not set up a country club; they make it tough on players to make the players prove themselves every day. If they can't take it, they go to the country-club teams or just to the country, out of baseball."

The crow said, "Why are you telling me all this? I got a family to keep, you know. I *know* it's tough."

"Exactly!" said the eagle. "It is tough simply to survive! Try now to understand what it takes to excel. Here goes Bob looking like gold. He has now married and has two kids. He works his way to the pinnacle of baseball, the New York Yankees, when in 1954 he comes to the Yankees from the Baltimore Orioles. You can look up his sports record.[†] He is called 'Bullet Bob" because of his fastball and, in 1955, he sets a record in his first year with the Yanks...in number of *walks!* Right there he could have quit...right then, but he and the managers saw that he also was fourth in strikeouts.

"Bob wants the pinnacle. He works to make himself get even better, and...ta da, in 1958 he is the hero of the World Series. That year he wins the Cy Young Award, The Sporting News 1958 Major League All Star Team and the American League Pitcher of the Year, the Baseball Writers Award, and the Hickock Belt as Top

Professional Athlete of the Year of *all* sports."

"Whoa! And Gawk!" said the crow. "He must have been in fat city."

"He wasn't fat," said the eagle.

"It's slang, eagle. What's the matter with you? I thought you was educated. It means he had a *huge* feather in his cap. But it hurts to think about that phrase. So now Bob lived happily ever after."

"Well," said the eagle. "As usual in life, it is difficult to repeat major success. The Yanks kept him on through 1962 and then shipped him off to the Angels and then the Angels dumped him, so he became a pitching coach for the Boston Red Sox. Obviously, this was a tough time and it resulted in his divorce also."

"So now he became a drunk on skid row," said the crow.

"Well, there are a lot of people who have been broken by becoming a has-been and who have buried themselves in drugs of some kind. What these people are saying to themselves is 'I really never deserved the attention I had. I always knew I was a failure.' Or they become bitter and blame the world for their lack of success. Yeah, Bob could have sunk to the bottom. In fact, the unhappiest day in his life was when the Yankees let him go without one word of gratitude for the years he put into the team. Bob could have said to himself that it wasn't his fault...that it was the stupid management."

"But he had vision. He knew better," said the crow.

"Well, you figure it out," said the eagle. "As pitching

coach at Boston, he was paid too little to cover his expenses, so he worked on the side for Hostess Cakes. But with his alimony and child support for two sons, he was still completely broke. He got another offer and he moved to Houston as a pitcher, but he soon discovered that he had no drive any longer. He could tell he wasn't really trying because he didn't even hurt after the game the way he used to. So then he went to Atlanta as a pitching coach taking an offer of $9,000 for the year."

"I swear," said the crow. "He must have been one miserable dude."

"Probably, but Bob never let himself get there. At the same time as he was pitching coach for Atlanta, he took a job selling bonds in a securities firm. He was up at 5:30 AM to sell securities. Then at 3:00 PM he was pitching coach until 1:00 AM. That is a twenty-hour day. But, already after one year, 1965, he earned $100,000."

"Gawk!" said the crow. "How did he do that?"

"Once again, I will explain. Bob did not sit and mope. He understood that his baseball career, which he had worked for and dreamed of his whole life, was over at age 35. But, Bob also understood that he needed to adapt and that he needed to work at something else. He knew he was not going to wait around for lady luck, because he knew that one makes his own luck. Things do not just come to you out of nowhere for no reason. Most people who play the lottery hope and believe that luck will happen to them. But, in real life, if you put everything you have into work, it results in economic success."

"Not if your boss sucks," said the crow.

"Ah, yes." The eagle paused for a moment to think just how to phrase the answer. This was a crucial point to get across to the crow, but also one of the most difficult. The eagle said slowly, "Bob did not choose to work for a boss. He had learned many positive things in baseball that he felt he could use for the rest of his life. And, in fact, he always wished everyone had been in sports to learn team spirit and cooperation. But he especially learned that he needed to be *in control*. He had suddenly become *old* in baseball, and, worst of all, baseball team management had been in complete control over his future...or lack thereof.

"He had previously learned that in the securities business, there is no salary. He could earn from his efforts. He could earn as much as he cared to work. All he needed to do was pick up the phone and talk to people. He knew what rejection was...something impersonal. It was part of the job. But he also knew what success felt like. He simply needed to work. Any *goofing off* and procrastination simply cost him income."

"So now, finally, he was in fat city," said the crow triumphantly.

"Almost," said the eagle.

"Almost! Gawk! Almost! I give up!" said the crow, and flew off.

The eagle sighed and said out loud, "I wonder if he will learn."

Chapter 4
Why Bother?

"I gotta know," said the crow the minute he landed. It took him a bit to get settled. He cleaned his beak and turned around on the branch a few times to get comfortable. "Didn't this guy ever have any fun?"

"Of course, and the stories are many," said the eagle. "One day on a mountain top we can relax and tell stories."

The crow seemed to be thinking. "What happened to this guy? I think you were about to tell me he sucked wind again. I'm afraid to hear it."

The eagle was pleased to see that the crow had settled in to listen. That was a good sign. "Well, to make a tough story short, after earning so well in the securities business, he bought into or outright bought some businesses...restaurants, a night club and a furniture factory. Of course, he really didn't have the money, so he borrowed deeply."

"But, at least, he was boss, right?" said the crow.

"Yeah, he was boss *and owner* all right." The eagle grimaced as only eagles can. "In 1972 the oil embargo had started and times were not good. A tornado comes in and rips one of his factories to smithereens. Then employees who, being the exact opposite of Bob, had decided that the world owed them something...went union. Bob couldn't afford it, so he sold one furniture factory.

"Then on a Sunday in June of 1973 a fire took his night club. Then immediately following Monday the bank came to his door and demanded that all notes be paid in seven days, not because of anything Bob had done, but because of changes in the banking regulations. He literally lost everything."

"Gawk."

"And he had personally signed all notes. It was about to become one of the biggest personal bankruptcies in Georgia."

"So he flew the coop," said the crow.

"Just the opposite. He refused to declare bankruptcy, which would erase his debt to the bank and the creditors. The court judge thought he was crazy for not declaring personal bankruptcy, but, since he wouldn't, Bob was given approval to declare Chapter 13 and to pay off his creditors. Bob paid them off in seven years."

"Why?" asked the crow.

Again the eagle sat in thought. It was another tough nut to crack. "This is the hardest lesson of all for winners. It is a combination of honesty, duty, and concern for society, which all adds up to *integrity*. Bob established that he had integrity back when he was a baseball pitcher. No matter how frustrated he had been...no matter what the coach might have requested, Bob refused to hit the batter with the ball on purpose. And therefore he had a second nickname of *Gentleman Bob*."

"It doesn't sound like it was a good idea taking on responsibility to pay off all his creditors when he didn't have to," said the crow.

"The integrity attitude is something only great leaders have and it gives returns a hundred-fold."

"I don't see how," said the crow. "He is obviously broke and paying out of his nose in alimony and child support."

"Yes, he is broke and he is jobless. Many people would give up at this point either by blaming the world or saying they couldn't get out from under such huge obligations. Bob, or anyone of integrity, does not see any other approach than telling himself that there is a way out."

"So, now it is time for the lottery," said the crow.

"So, now it is time for work. Bob searched the newspapers for a job where, if he worked, he could earn from his effort. He didn't look for a salaried job; he needed to earn good money. He knew a little about investing from his previous work so, when he saw a sales job for insurance, he decided that he should sell life insurance."

"Life insurance is investing?"

"Bob had in his mind to sell life insurance a special way.

Instead of selling *whole* life insurance policies the way the insurance companies had been doing, his principled mind said he should sell *term* life insurance, which was cheap, and explain to his clients how to invest the difference in the stock market, particularly mutual funds."

"I don't understand," said the crow.

"It was quite simple, although revolutionary. Bob knew that for the same money that a family would normally put into whole life insurance (and which simply went into the coffers of the insurance companies, even though they said it was an investment), his customers could put just a little piece of *that* money into term insurance (with *more* insurance protection than the whole life) and put the remaining money into mutual funds, which really were investments."

"That makes sense," said the crow. "But why hadn't everyone already done that?"

"Quite simply because the insurance companies didn't guide their salesmen to do that, because the companies made *much* more money on whole life insurance. Also, because it was a harder sell, the companies offered their salesmen a higher commission on whole life to make it more attractive to the sales rep."

"So Bob should have done that. He needed the money."

"He needed it badly. And he was willing to work for it. But Gentleman Bob, Mr. Integrity couldn't cheat people. Besides, he did earn money on selling term insurance and he also made money on the mutual funds."

"So everybody was happy," said the crow.

"So everybody was not happy," said the eagle.

"Gawk! What now?"

"Bob did so well selling term insurance that the insurance company he represented asked him to stop doing it."

"Huh?"

"He was literally ruining the whole life business for the insurance company. So he moved to another insurance company and, after a while, they, too, said the same thing. So he went to a third company and once again caught gaff for selling term insurance. After five years of struggling with having too much success in the *wrong* area with these insurance companies, Bob went hunting for a firm that would like him to sell term insurance. He helped found a new company with a fellow called Art Williams. This became A.L. Williams Insurance, which later changed its name to Primerica. This company became so successful that it bought Travelers Insurance which later merged with City Corp to become City Group."

"Well, that was easy," said the crow.

"It was about as easy as pushing a battleship backwards with your bare hands."

"Gawk! What are you talking about?"

"The insurance companies hated A.L. Williams Insurance Company once they realized the impact of this new company. The existing insurance companies and the insurance industry used every dirty trick in their arsenal to bury this company."

"How?" said the crow.

"In ways too numerous to count, but generally by producing bad publicity, siccing the insurance commissioners on A.L. Williams, and having their reps tell tall tales, which, of course, wasn't too difficult since they were trained in it."

"And what happened?"

"Each time the Insurance Commission checked out A.L. Williams Insurance, A.L. Williams was lauded for its policies and honesty. Bob's part of the business grew and grew and grew and is still growing all over America and Canada, with world expansion in the offing. Bob is able to trade homes as a hobby and to live at an economic level few people in the world have attained."

"How did that happen?"

"Remember. I said that integrity comes back to you in big ways. Customers recognized Bob's integrity and wanted to deal with him despite what the big, existing insurance companies said. And people wanted to work with Bob because they felt his integrity. And Bob knew what it took to make a viable company...help everyone who works with you to have success. This was not easy. It is never easy to be successful."

"So everyone can be successful?"

"You! You, Crow, need to answer that question for yourself. There is room for everyone to be successful...to become eagles."

"Gawk!" said the crow and flew away.

The eagle sighed. He had probably said the wrong thing.

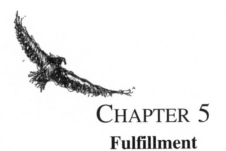

CHAPTER 5
Fulfillment

"You made me angry yesterday," said the crow. The eagle said nothing. "You suggested that a crow is not as good as an eagle." Again, the eagle said nothing. The crow flew down to a lower branch and back up again. Then he circled the tree, landed on the lower branch, and then flapped up again. After another pause, he said, "You *were* a crow, weren't you?"

"Yes," said the eagle.

"In fact, you are the same Bob as in the story, aren't you?" The eagle was silent. "You are his soul." Both birds sat bobbing on their branches looking out over the beautiful earth. As if thinking out loud, the crow said, "I am the soul of someone somewhere." He looked at the eagle waiting for a response.

"Yes, you are," said the eagle.

The crow was silent for a while, seemingly thinking. "Are you happy?" asked the crow.

"Happy is not a choice. Happiness is a temporary state often dependent on present circumstances...marriage, children, friends, and other outside influences. Happiness is not so much having what you want, as wanting what you have.[3] It is not something that you can control and it is extremely relative to one's previous experience."

"So why bother?" said the crow. "I don't see the point of all this work and integrity if you can't be happy."

"I didn't say a successful person cannot be happy. In fact, he can be as happy as the next person at any one time. But a successful person is *fulfilled*. *Fulfillment* is a gradual process like the growth of this oak in which we are sitting."

The crow interrupted. "This is NOT an oak. This is an elm!"

"I told you trees are not my strong suit. *Mountains* are. Anyway, it takes ages for an elm to get to this size, but once it does, it is solid and visible. *Fulfillment* is strong and visible because *fulfillment* brings contentment and confidence."

"It sounds like a religion," said the crow.

"That is exactly what religion is based on...giving people a fulfillment."

"But this tree can be chopped down," said the crow.

"This tree can very much be chopped down," said the eagle. "Just as integrity...and the *fulfillment* thereof...can be lost. So once the strength of *fulfillment* is felt, one can not stop treating others with respect and helping others to be successful."

The crow looked at the eagle. He looked at his proud head and his massive wings. And then he said, "And that is why

[3] Hyman Schachtel

you are talking to me."

"That is why I am talking to you," said the eagle. "I know that you are an uncommon crow. You have something special in you, I think."

"How do you know?" asked the crow.

"A little birdie told me. But I can do no more than *tell* you that. I can only tell you about the possibilities, as your parents did about flying. I have spoken to thousands of crows...all of whom I thought were possible eagles, but many are still crows like those squawking over in the road there. They find it far too difficult to take the responsibility of living a life of integrity. They simply tell themselves that they are not capable...that they are not worth it."

The crow was intently watching the crows fighting over road-kill. He said, "But some crows have become eagles?"

"Yes. They have." The eagle watched the crow. Finally, without making a peep, the crow flew off into the distance.

The eagle sighed and thought about what plan to follow next. Should he search for another crow right now? Should he take a trip to see his family? Should he visit with his new eagle friends? "Crow-knees" he called them. Maybe he should remind them that neither he nor they must ever stop looking for crows to support.

For the moment, however, he decided that he would just soar for a while and enjoy the earth. He needed that, too.

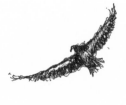

Chapter 6

Above It All

From Bob's position, he had a bird's-eye view of the area...his area. He felt an affinity for it...almost a love. He knew it partly had to do with ego, but he knew ego is a frailty. Ego is something that can be corrupted, manipulated, and controlled by others and must never be the dominant force for any decision. Baseball had taught him that. And he was particular about point-ing out the peacock, which has such fine feathers, but has nothing to offer the rest of society. The peacock needs its fine feathers to hide its insecurities and it bores others with its self-occupation. He had seen eagles transform into peacocks to then damage what they had built.

Bob's past experience had put him in such turbulence that even the birds were walking. But he knew he could not tell others how to live their lives. At a young age he had become a wily old bird. Even as a young baseball player, he once said, "The only way you can get people to follow you is to lead by your own principles and then people will follow you if they like you."

Right now, while soaring in the heavens, he had to chuckle, as only eagles can do, when he thought back on his eagle-eye ability. Back in his earliest career with the Saint Louis Browns, which at that time was the worst team in the league, rather than be depressed and bored by the losing, Bob occupied himself by studying the opposing pitchers. And he discovered that he could read their body language so well that he could discern, to a high degree, what ball they were about to pitch at any one time.

He developed this ability to such a degree that, when Bob came to the Yankees, this ability could be exploitable as an offensive batting system. To improve their hitting, Mickey Mantle and Gil McDougald, especially, worked with Bob to read the opposing pitchers, using a secret whistling system. It had to be secret, not only so that the opposing team wouldn't catch on, but also, even within the Yankees, Bob knew some of the players might be traded and would then expose the secret to other teams.

Bob would read the pitcher's windup and then, having developed a whistle that could be heard above the crowd, he signaled to Mickey or Gil. They, on their part, could signal back with hand jesters to ask for confirmation or repeats. In some cases, because of certain pitchers' obvious movement or placement on the rubber, Bob could teach Mickey or Gil how to read the pitcher without Bob's signals, which helped preserve the secret.

His eagle-eyed ability to observe the body language of others continued to help him deal with people in general. It was a talent that he could not teach, but as with flying, he could let his adherents know of the powers of observation. It gave him great satisfaction to help others to gain economic success. Coaching baseball had a certain satisfaction, but had two inherent problems: 1) it paid too little for him to survive and 2) the recipient, as with Bob himself, would only be successful as long as his body and his will held up. In Bob's financial business experience, he saw how 1) he could earn a living and 2) help others to have a life-time of financial security and comfort.

Looking over his realm, he knew it was only four-in-twenty blackbirds that might be able to conceive of becoming an eagle. He knew he needed to continue to recruit since a bird in the hand was certainly NOT worth two working in the bush. Suddenly his eagle eye caught a glimpse of something that could only warm his heart.

There in the tallest oak (or was it an elm?) was Gawk... molting... shedding his crow's feathers. He was intently talking with a crow, which was nervously hopping from one branch to another. Bob knew Gawk did not want anyone to disrupt. Gawk had become a leader on his own. So Bob let out his signature strong whistle. Gawk got the signal.

PART TWO
Visits

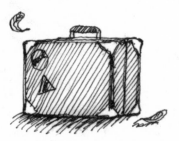

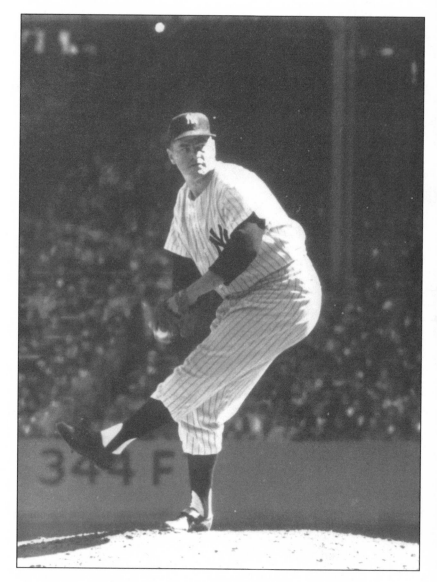

Bob Turley pitching in Yankee's uniform

Gawking on "The Mound"

When he had time, Gawk did come to Bob's mountain, which, of course, Bob called "The Mound." Gawk wanted to talk with a winner. Here are random outtakes of those conversations (be aware that Gawk is no longer a crow, but crow thinking has been added here for analysis).

ABOUT TODAY'S PLAYERS: **When I grew up, once you signed a contract with a team, you were their property for life. So it was almost like slavery. I suppose that, if we wanted to make a big enough stink about it, we could have gotten off a team. And some guys do that today. But the ballplayer today is, in my opinion, a better ball player from a standpoint of the physical. Roger Clemens, 38 or 39 years old, still winning twenty games and almost striking out 300 guys every year is unreal. But, of course, they can do it as a living year round and don't have to go home in the winter to work and make a living.**

Crow's View: They should have been unionized.

Eagle's View: I make the best of my present situation, although I need to be in control of my future.

ABOUT BASEBALL: It was every young man's dream to be in the major leagues, but you couldn't make any money to retire on. We went in for the recognition. We never even thought about the money part of it until later. But most of the guys played the game just because they liked it.

Crow's View: I wouldn't want to take that chance.

Eagle's View: If I do something for the love of it, something good will always come out of it.

ABOUT CAREER LOWS: I was traded twice. The first one enhanced my life tremendously. I was traded up to the New York Yankees. The second trade, Roy Hamey, the General Manager of the New York Yankees, notified me that they had traded me to Los Angeles after eight years with the Yankees...with a slip in a hotel message box. No one ever called me. It was the lowest point in my life. It was like my whole world exploded.

Crow's View: They will do it to you every time.

Eagle's View: I don't have time to mope about. I learn something from every situation and I pull up those proverbial bootstraps.

ON BOUNCING BACK: If it's baseball, you can't win every game or strike out every hitter. In sales you can't close every deal. In baseball I had to wait four days before I could do it again. At least, in business I can immediately go at it again. And I always have something to look forward to, all the time.

Crow's View: I hate when I make a fool of myself, so I need more training and personal help until I know how to sell.

Eagle's View: Who is next? I know I will have success next time.

ABOUT PITCHERS: When I got the pitching coach job with the Boston Red Sox, I called Jim, the pitching coach for the Yankees, and said, "We are going to have a big pitching camp. Jim, what the devil do you do with all these guys?" He said, "Bob, it is very simple. When you get to the spring training, have a meeting with your guys and say, 'Gentlemen, this is the mound; this is a baseball; here is the baseball; go at it.' Bob, you don't have to do anything. They will show you what they can do. You will know who has the most talent and who are the best ones."

Crow's View: I can't handle this. I will get eaten alive.

Eagle's View: I'll just do it and see what I can learn.

ABOUT THE BOSTON RED SOX: Well, when I was there, the manager was Mr. All-American Johnny Pesky. He was a great ball player for the Red Sox and everybody loved him. He was one of those that you just wanted to cuddle. Johnny was a good person, but he had a problem with Mike Higgins, who was the General Manager of the ball club. For example, one year we were playing without a full team because of injuries and players sent down to the minor leagues. We certainly did *not* have enough pitchers. I was there when Johnny called Mike Higgins. Higgins said he was going out to Portland, Oregon, to scout a pitcher named Joey Jay. It sounded a little fishy because Joey Jay had been in the Boston Red Sox organization for six to eight years previously. So by now you would think Mike Higgins knew the guy. One day went by. Two days went by. Three days went by. Mike Higgins never called Johnny Pesky. Mike Higgins had gone on a fishing trip out in Portland. Real fish.

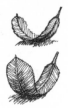

Crow's View: I can't depend on anybody.

Eagle's View: I have to be aware of what is going on in all areas of my business at all times so I can compensate for weaknesses.

ABOUT THE WILD LIFE: When I was out in Hollywood during my first training camp, three of us were fixed up with blind dates. We were all kinds of cocky. We told a big story about how we were major league ball players (even though we were still minor league). One of the girls said that we should go the Macombo which was a big entertainment place. And, sure enough, there's Tyrone Powers and his wife Christine sitting there. And over there is Jack Benny. I said, "Oh, my god. We ain't got any money." All we got was $25 a week for laundry. All three of us together had $75 on us.

So we go into this club, all of us guys feigning lack of hunger and I drink a Coke. When they brought us the check, it was for $73. I'll always remember that. When we paid, I grabbed the change. When the parking attendant brought our car around, it cost two dollars, without tip. After a dirty look from the attendant, we headed for home when one of the girls wanted to go into this famous drug store where Lana Turner was discovered. After we got in there, because we had no money, we three told the girls that we had to run back because of curfew or we would be fined $100. So we left the girls there and, needless to say, that was the last we saw of them.

Crow's View: It is just the rich and famous who have fun.

Eagle's View: What great fun and great memories I have had.

THE EARLY YEARS: The second year in the minors, I got a $600 bonus with which I bought a Model A Ford. But as a ball club we rode in an old yellow school bus with the manager as the driver. If the bus broke down, we would sleep on the bus. Most of the trips weren't very long, but I remember going to Marian, Illinois, to play in the Illinois State League. Going back to the hotel we found all our bags waiting outside the hotel because the club hadn't paid the rent. It was another night of sleeping on the bus. Once in the summer, we robbed a watermelon patch and escaped in the bus. Our meal allowance was $1.75 per day.

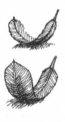

Crow's View: What a *sucky* time! I couldn't live under such circumstances.

Eagle's View: I had so much fun and comradery that it has lasted me a lifetime.

A HORSE SHOOT: There were lots of stories about Mickey Mantle, Billy Martin, and Whitey Ford shooting a horse. One of the stories goes that Mickey was going to play a practical joke on his buddies. So having permission to hunt on a farmer's land, the farmer asks Mickey to shoot an old nag while he is there. So Mickey didn't tell the other guys about the request. When they get to the farm, Mickey says something like 'Watch this,' and shoots the horse. Supposedly, the other guys then decide to shoot the rest of the livestock. Or another versions tells of Billy Martin shooting the horse and then Mickey shooting another. None of this is true, but it made for a funny story.

Crow's View: What could I possibly learn from this?

Eagle's View: Nothing, but it is a fun story that is so widespread that a correction is needed.

THE BOSTON RED SOX: Johnny Pesky told the team one night, "Look, fellas, we're in contention here. We have to get our rest tonight. I want everybody in their rooms in an hour and a half." So nobody pays any attention. Only one out of twenty-five was in his room. So the next day at a clubhouse meeting, Johnny said, "I asked you to be in your rooms. You disobeyed, so now you are fined. You'll get your notices soon." Higgins is still out fishing in Portland, Oregon, so Johnny tells Yawkey, the owner, about the fines. Yawkey politely proceeded the next day to cancel all the fines. Everything was undermined in that organization. I've never seen so many guys with so much talent, but could never win. Winning wasn't that important to them from my point of view.

Crow's View: I wouldn't go tell the owner. Talk about backstabbing.

Eagle's View: My integrity does not stop me from acting in a proper fashion even if I know those around me may be lacking. It is obvious to me that it takes support from the top down to make a winning team.

RED SOX MANAGEMENT: We just finished a series in Boston and we had flown to California. I was sitting in the hotel lobby about three in the morning waiting for my luggage. A newspaper reporter named Henry McKenna, who was a great fan of Boston, sat beside me and said, "Let me ask you something. What's wrong with the Red Sox? Why can't they win?" I tell him it's not my position to tell him. He said, "Hey, Bob, I'm not going to write anything. I'm just a great fan and whatever you say is between us. I'm not going to write anything." So like a dumb, young, pitching coach, I politely told him what I thought was wrong with the club. He immediately went to another writer and told him the story. After that, I knew I was in trouble for sure. I went in to Tom Yawkey and apologized. Typically, Tom Yawkey says, "Bob, I understand. You weren't doing anything to hurt anybody. You were just having a private conversation. No problem." A good owner would have fired my ass right on the spot.

Crow's View: I think it is great to be forgiven for a rookie mistake.

Eagle's View: Although I am aware of the mistake I made, the leniency shown me does not inspire me. And it certainly does not inspire the rest of the team.

On Winning: The difference between a losing ball club and a winning ball club is so small. It's all attitude. The Yankees paid a lot of guys pretty good money who never hit much. But these guys did a lot to make the club win. I've seen Hank Bauer go up to the plate in the late innings at the end of September and stay up there to let a ball hit him with the bases loaded. But I have seen other guys in the major leagues in the same situation jump and fall back, and then raise hell with the pitcher. All they *needed* to do was let the ball nick them and the game was won.

Crow's View: I don't see the point of sacrificing myself. Let somebody else do it.

Eagle's View: I will follow closely every aspect of what it takes to win and make sure that I try to do my part.

ON WINNING INTENTIONS: There was a ball player by the name of Joe Peppertone who had good ability. I mean, great ability. He played in the major leagues a long time, but Joe loved to be liked. I guess he still does today, but we were trying to win ball games. Joe would come on the field but never give his best. He was not playing a team sport with us. Even though he was hitting over 300 and twenty home runs, we didn't want him on our ball club. His intentions were not to win. In baseball as in business, you have to be involved in every part of it. If a person doesn't have the winning attitude, doesn't want to win, I don't care if you are in baseball or business, you are not going very far.

 Crow's View: I'm doing my part. Look at my statistics. I can't help it if others can't match my results.

 Eagle's View: Not everyone is capable of just what I do, but they have other strengths. I need everyone's strengths in order for me and my team to win. I need to see what I can do to help them.

MICKEY MANTLE: He would do anything to win. I watched Mickey in the late innings bunt, get to first base, steal second, steal third, and score on a ground ball to win the game. He loved to win more than anything else. He loved to hit the baseball, but winning was more important. Roger Maris was the same.

 Crow's View: Some people have all the talent.

 Eagle's View: I truly admire those who make themselves winners by thinking what more they can do and by making an effort in every facet.

ON PITCHING: **There are dumb pitchers and there are good pitchers. Dumb pitchers just throw everything the catcher says. That tells you he is not even thinking about the game. Good pitchers know what they are going to do. For example, when I pitched Bob Allison, who hit a lot of home runs for the Minnesota Twins, he never got any hits off me. I knew he was looking for the fastball right down the middle because I was a fastball pitcher. So the first pitch I would throw a fastball up high. Ball one. Then I would throw a curve ball down on the ground. Ball two. Now he is sure I am going to throw a fastball, but I would throw a high slider that looks like a fastball, but it breaks the last second. The best he did was hit a nice soft fly to the center field. I pitched him my whole career that way and he never realized what I was doing. A catcher can't do that for you.**

Crow's View: I'm not the one who is supposed to do that job. Let the specialist figure it out.

Eagle's View: If, by having control, I can improve the winning chances, I am going to take responsibility.

Whitey Ford: Whitey Ford called his own games. It wasn't that Yogi Berra wasn't smart; he was probably the best there ever was. But he is looking at the ball like a hitter; the pitcher sees it as it is going towards home. Whitey used to bend over when he was going to throw a fastball, so the infielders knew what was coming. If he shook his glove, it was a curve ball. If he wanted to start all over and reverse it, he rubbed across his chest or stood up.

Crow's View: Why bother making a fool of myself? I might make a mistake. I've got the job already.

Eagle's View: What actions can I take to improve the situation so as to benefit the team and make us all winners?

On Baseball and Business: You have got to think ahead and plan like a pitcher does. But, if you are just going to do what everybody else is doing, you aren't going anywhere. You have got to be a little bit different. You have got to be a little bit more aggressive. That is why I keep calling on all my baseball experience, because it relates so well to the business world.

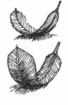

Crow's View: I ain't sticking my neck out.

Eagle's View: Is there any action I can take that is even better than what has been done before?

ON BUSINESS: I have sat and talked to guys that are very intelligent and make a lot of money. Listening to them talk about their businesses, and because of their attitude, they make it sound easy. I don't care what the product is, it isn't any good unless you can get it on the market. I kept it simple. We just made people feel fantastic about this great company. It was very difficult to duplicate what we were doing because we were doing it with enthusiasm and we were doing it from the bottom of the scale all the way to the top. Everybody was excited and pulling together as a team. The end result, we all came out winners.

Crow's View: The big guys are smarter than I am and they don't have time for me. They will only take advantage of me.

Eagle's View: What can I learn from talking to winners? How do they inspire others to want to win?

ON DELEGATING: You have a son and he wants to try the power mower to cut the grass. You are a little skeptical, but one day you say okay. He gets out there and cuts the grass. When you come out to look, you see spots all over that he missed and all kinds of problems. You have two choices at that moment. You can point out all the faults or you can say what a great job he has done. "Fantastic. I can't believe you cut the grass. You must have cut grass before." You know what will happen. The next time it will be better.

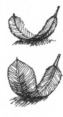

Crow's View: I don't have time to make up for other's mistakes.

Eagle's View: What can I do to help his person improve his performance and make it rewarding?

ON EGO: I have seen egoists that wore their egos on a cuff-link. When people under them started making a lot of money and almost making as much money as these people, these egomaniacs got so damn jealous that they then drove the moneymakers right out of the business.

Crow's View: I don't want anybody making a fool of me. I'm the boss.

Eagle's View: How great it would be if my underlings could do better than I ever did and hatch into major winners. Then I know we all win.

ON OPPORTUNITY: I had a lot of guys from the baseball world, football world, basketball world call and want to come to work with me. We spent time talking. I told them, if you know what you are doing, you can make more money than you will ever make otherwise. The one thing that stopped them from coming to work with me was that they wanted to know what my guarantees were. I said there are no guarantees.

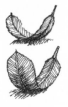

Crow's View: I've got to know what I am going to get paid.

Eagle's View: Please don't limit my possibilities.

ON GUIDANCE: I would tell my people that maybe it is uncomfortable for you to talk to me, but don't you ever lie to me because I can't help a person that will lie to me about a situation. Tell me the truth and we can solve the problem and probably save time. But you have people whose truth is their truth. It is the way they see it and I don't call that a lie.

Crow's View: You can't really trust what people say.

Eagle's View: Everybody has a viewpoint. Let's figure out how to make it all work.

ON LEARNING: When I came to the major leagues, I wanted to talk to anyone that would give me the knowledge that could enhance my training and experience. I wouldn't talk to the five-and-twenty-five pitcher, but I would talk to a pitcher that was fifteen and five. Just ask them a question, and most good people in baseball and in business everywhere are willing to share. They are not afraid of losing a job to you. And it makes them feel good to give.

Crow's View: Everybody has his own agenda and they are probably out to screw me. Besides, as I have always said, they don't have time for me.

Eagle's View: Who are the winners that can and want to help me succeed? I want to talk to them.

ON TAKING ACTION: When I signed my first contract in 1948 on June 15th and got out of high school, I went to play professional baseball. I had never played anything except muni-league ball and high school ball, where I knew a lot of the people. Now I was headed to a strange team. I didn't know a soul. How could I survive in the surroundings of these guys who are such heroes to me and that I am in such awe of? There I was on the mound, *facing* these heroes. But I threw a couple of pitches and very quickly I got more confident because, hell, they couldn't hit me any better than the kids in high school.

Crow's View: I'm not good enough.

Eagle's View: I'm probably never good enough, but I am going to find out how good I am and what I can do to improve.

ON SELLING: To be successful in sales, it is important to read the client as you speak, and most importantly, you have got to be a hell of a good listener.

Crow's View: People don't really want me to be selling them something.

Eagle's View: Life is selling. The better I can figure out what people want, the better it will be for both of us.

ON WEALTHY EGO: **Some people make a lot of money, but still no one knows who they are. There are two ways to go. Go into politics or buy a major league sports team. But owners who have not played the sport are not usually successful owners.**

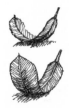

Crow's View: I need to buy something that will show my worth.

Eagle's View: I need to do what I love to do.

ON BRAVADO: **Don't oversell yourself. You just go out and do your job, pay attention to your job, and improve yourself.**

Crow's View: Look at *me*!

Eagle's View: What can I do to better myself?

ON SUCCESS: I didn't play on all good teams and I didn't play on all bad teams. But with experience, I could see the difference between good teams and bad teams and, after a while, I could understand why they were good and why they were bad. It did not have to do with ability.

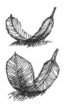

Crow's View: I know I'm not as good as you are, so don't expect much.

Eagle's View: What can I do to help us win?

ON DRIVE: Most people who want to be successful, in 90% of the cases, it is because a parent, a brother or sister, or former employee told them that they would never make it. And they want to be successful to prove to everybody that they were wrong.

Crow's View: I don't know anybody who believes I can do it. All my friends tell me that it is stupid to try.

Eagle's View: I know I can exceed and become successful despite when other people try to drag me down to their level. I know misery loves company. I fear being mediocre. I love the feeling of success.

ON LIFE: I say that the way to ruin your life is to worry about something that you can't change.

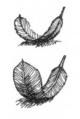

Crow's View: I can't believe they did that to me.

Eagle's View: What's next? Wow! Look at those possibilities!

And just before Gawk flew off the other day, he said to Bob, "You know what I discovered?"

"What's that?" asked Bob.

"I'm nobody special and yet I am so far ahead of my old friends. Winning is 90% attitude and 10% ability. It makes me feel so good to be successful."

"Amen," said Bob.

The End

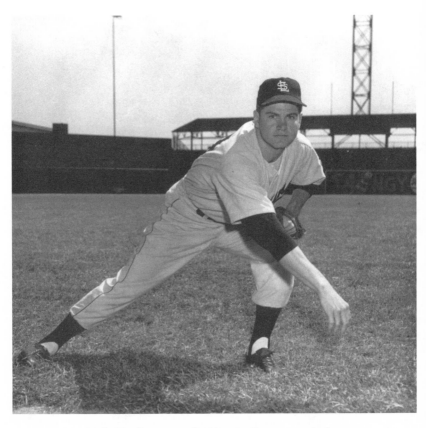

Bob Turley as a St. Louis Browns pitcher

About Bob Turley

† From *The Yankee Encyclopedia*

Turley, Bob
Nickname: "Bullet Bob"
Pitcher
Born: September 19, 1930
Birthplace: Troy, Ill
Bat: R Throw: R
Ht: 6' 2" Wt: 215

Honors: In 1958 Bob won the Cy Young Memorial Award as the best pitcher in the Major Leagues. *The Sporting News* selected Bob as the American League Pitcher of the Year and the Major League Player of the Year in 1958, and the Baseball Writers gave Bob the Sid Mercer Award. He also won the Hickok Belt as the Top Professional Athlete of the Year in 1958, and *The Sporting News* selected him as one of three pitchers on the publication's 1958 Major League All-Star team.

Came to Yanks: In November 1954, Bob came to the Yanks from the Baltimore Orioles as part of an eighteen-player trade, the largest trade in Major League history.

Fastball Pitcher: "Bullet Bob" possessed a scorching, lively fastball and, when he was on the top of his game (as he was during the entire 1958 season), Bob was as tough to hit as any pitcher in history. Mickey Mantle stated he never saw a harder thrower than Bob when he was right. Bob had a good curveball, but he used it as his waste pitch and for setting up batters. To be effective in a game, Bob needed his blazing fastball and a lot of strikeouts indicating he had his speed. Sometimes Bob was wild. In 1955 he walked 177 batters, the most ever by a Yankee right-hander, and he led the American League in walks in 1955 and 1958 (128). Only four times has a Yankee pitcher recorded more strikeouts than Bob's 210 in 1955. For his Major League career, Bob allowed only 7.18 hits per nine innings, the eighth best ratio in Major League history. Bob got his childhood pitching practice throwing pears in his back yard.

Yankee Star: As a Yankee pitcher, Bob hurled three one-hitters, tying him with Whitey Ford for the most in Yankee history. In his best Yankee seasons (1955, 1958), he was the Yank's ace starter. He was the club's third starter in 1956 and the second starter in 1957. In the 1959 Yankee Stadium home opener, Bob beat the Red Sox, 3-2, but his 8-11 record in 1959 was disappointing on the heels of his splendid 1958 season. Bob and Whitey Ford teamed to form an excellent right-left combination for the Yanks in the late 1950's. In 1960 Bob was the Yanks' third starter and although his 9-3 record was not sensational, the Yanks won 14 of the 15 games in which he was relieved after starting. A sore arm ruined his 1961 campaign. He attempted to pitch with constant arm pain, but finally was placed on the disabled list for much of the season, then had surgery. He was used mostly in relief in 1962.

Fine Gentleman: Although Bob's fastball was frighteningly quick, batters were not usually intimidated because they knew that Bob was too much of a gentleman to throw at a hitter. On the Yanks, he was known as a serious, religious fellow, but one who was quite friendly and liked by his teammates. There was one bit of deception, though, at which Bob was especially adept. He could discover telltale signs in other pitchers that allowed him to know what kind of pitch was to be delivered. As soon as he learned the pitch, Bob quickly relayed the information (usually by whistling) to the Yankee batter who gained a great advantage. Mickey Mantle hit many home runs after being tipped by Bob.

League Leader: In 1958, Bob led American League pitchers in wins, winning percentage (21-7, .750) and complete games (19).

Club Leadership: Besides his American League leading stats in 1958, Bob also led the Yanks in innings pitched (245). Three times he led the Yanks in strikeouts and shutouts. Bob led the club in complete games in two straight seasons (1957-1958). Twice he led the team in games started.

All-Time Yankee Leader: Bob is tenth on the all-time Yankee shutout list (21). He is eleventh on the all-time Yankee strikeout list (909).

All-Star Game: Bob was selected to the American League team for the 1955 and 1958 All-Star games. He started the 1958 All-Star Game.

World Series: In game six of the 1956 series, Bob fanned eleven Dodgers, the most ever recorded by a losing pitcher in a World Series game. Bob lost a 1-0 heartbreaker in the tenth inning when a ball was misplayed in the outfield. In game six of the 1957 series, he pitched a four-hitter to beat Milwaukee, 3-2. Bob was the hero of the 1958 series, winning *Sport Magazine's* MVP Award. With the Yanks trailing three games to one, Bob kept the Yanks alive by blanking the Braves seven-zero in game 5. He returned in game six in relief to get the final Brave out, recording a save. Then in game seven, Bob won again, six-two, to give the Yanks a remarkable series comeback conquest. In game two of the 1960 series, he beat Pittsburgh, 16-3.

Left Yanks: Following the 1962 season, the Yanks sold Bob's contract to the Los Angeles Angels. In 1963 Bob was 2-7 for the Angels and 1-4 for the Red Sox in his last Major League season.